Close to Zero

Waste

Imperfectly perfect at

sustainability

Salinda Strandberg

This book is dedicated to my husband, Van, who supports any idea or decision I make.

To my mom, Malinda, for encouraging my "why" mentality and helping me learn to find the answers.

And to my children, Braxton, Tayah and Justin, who I want to leave a better world for.

Table of Contents

Contents

Chapter One 4

Chapter Two 16

Chapter Three.. 24

Chapter Four 35

Chapter Five 46

Chapter Six.. 71

Chapter Seven.. 85

Chapter Eight... 93

Chapter Nine.. 98

Chapter ten 115

From the Kitchen........................... 127

From the Bathroom 128

From the Laundry Room................... 128

From the Office............................... 129

Other Areas Around the House......... 129

Party and Holiday Supplies.............. 130

Pet-Related 130

"Unless someone like you cares a whole awful lot, nothing is going to get better. It's not" -The Lorax, Dr. Seuss

Chapter One

Introduction

"No one cares how much you know, until they know how much you care."- Theodore Roosevelt

There are thousands of zero waste books you could have chosen. Zero waste at home, zero waste on travel, zero waste at work, zero waste (insert location). This book is not an all-encompassing book, it's not a reference book, this book isn't even going to get you all the way to zero. This book is just a jumping off point. Something to help you reduce your current waste creation and simple ways to get there. This book isn't a list of ways to do it, it's more of a why and how to do it and you figure out where you want to make the changes.

My goal with this book is that you find it helpful, useful, but above all else, that you feel empowered to do something different. I want you to understand why you need to do something. That no matter how small you think it is, it's going to help. But, I really want you to feel something. I want this book to wake you up to how you can make a difference even in a world where we think that one person doesn't really matter all that much. I want you to know how much I care and that every little bit will help, I promise!

There are a ton of other zero waste books on Amazon, in the bookstores or at the library so why another zero-waste book you may ask. I'd like to say it's because I have all new information or that I have discovered the magic bullet to fix climate change; but neither of those is particularly true. I chose to write this book because I have felt from time to time that zero waste is too complicated to do and even I, who is overly passionate about the environment and what I can do (just ask my husband), find it hard to see how I can make a difference. So, I am writing this book to help those like me, who think it's not possible to reach zero waste.

Not to mention the tons of people over the last few decades that have told me things like **"zero waste just isn't possible for my family"**. I recycle, isn't that enough? **How can you have only a mason jar full of trash at the end of a year?** Who can just live off the land? **Who lives close enough to work, stores, friends, and family to only ride a bike every day and everywhere?** It's too radical of a lifestyle change. And my favorite, **"what can one person really do?"**

My answer is YES, it is radical going zero waste, but it is POSSIBLE to find a middle ground where you can reduce your footprint on the world and still maintain a healthy lifestyle. I'm not going to say you have to live in a tiny home on some small plot of land and only have 100 items to your name. If you do, that's cool! I'm not going to say you have to give up meat and become a vegan (if you want to do that after reading this or watching some documentaries, that's marvelous!). I'm not going to tell you that you HAVE to get solar panels on your house and drive an electric vehicle and never use plastics again. I'm just asking you to have an open mind as you read this book.

As for my favorite excuse "What can one person do?" A LOT!!

Think back into your childhood, is there a teacher, a neighbor, or a friend that changed you in some way? The answer is probably yes! They were just one person lending a hand or an ear for someone else. That help then allowed them to use the knowledge, wisdom, or compassion they learned to help at least one more person. Stanley Gordan West said it best, "Smile and the whole world smiles with you."

While we like to think we live in a bubble and that what we do doesn't really affect anyone else, the truth is we are all interconnected.

A few quick examples of how interconnected we are: A favorite game of mine, six degrees of separation, where we are all in some way connected to everyone else. I am one degree separation from Ryan Reynolds, but I don't remember getting a LinkedIn invite. I was in high school my freshman year with high school senior Richard Ruccolo and we were both in the school play. He even signed my program at the after party. Rich was in *Two Guys, a Girl, and a Pizza Place* with Ryan Reynolds.

Or on a more daily note, someone's bad mood can affect your day. Having that one coworker that snickered at your outfit can make you self-conscious all day.

Overall, I don't hunt but I eat meat. I don't farm but I eat corn. I don't bake bread but there's a loaf of it in my pantry. I didn't do any of those things, but I benefit from others doing those things. Why? Because we are interconnected and global.

On a larger scale, the pollution from India does make its way to America. The trash floating in the middle of the Pacific Ocean, "The Pacific Garbage Patch", comes from all over the world, as does the trash on the shores of any uninhabited islands.

But isn't it too late to make it matter? The temperature is rising, the ocean glaciers are melting, the summers start sooner, are hotter, and last longer. We don't see snow packed mountain peaks like we used to. Drought is becoming so familiar on the news that we can't even name just one spot where it's happening. Thousand years floods are happening every hundred years and Hundred-year floods are happening every decade. Miami is lifting their roads because they flood daily at high tide.

Mountain ski lodges are making fake snow so we can still ski and snowboard. All of this is true with the exception of one thing...it is never too late to make a change.

"Do something now. If not here, where? If not now, when? If not you, who?" - Theodore Roosevelt

Whatever parts of this book you decide to do or try, keep only what is sustainable for you. Like a new fad diet that comes out every year, most of them aren't sustainable. Starving yourself with no carbs, or eating like the cavemen, drinking all your calories, none of that can last forever. At some point you are going to feel like you are being too restrictive and no longer enjoying life. You are denying yourself all the things that make life worth living. You won't want to continue; you'll give up or you'll try a new one to see if that one will stick. The cycle will just continue. With this book, I want you to feel complete while making some changes that won't break the bank or your will to live.

Close to zero (low) waste is a lifestyle change not one of those fad consumers diets, like those "no buy" months that are celebrated. We have to find that balance between producing less waste (we will always make some sort of waste) and still being able to live.

The richest country in the world (United States of America) makes up 4.25% of the world's population and yet we produce over 4 times that of other world citizens in waste[1]. We are rich in not just money, but in freedoms...freedom of movement and

---

[1] Average American Carbon Footprint. Inspire Clean Energy.
https://www.inspirecleanenergy.com/blog/clean-energy-101/average-american-carbon-footprint#fnref1

that movement allows us to go, do, and be what we want. One of the things we should want to do is to leave a planet and natural resources for our future generations. We should want to be a steward for this planet. Like the man who plants a tree seed, the shade is not for him. He will never rest in the afternoon shade of that tree, but his grandchildren will.

I've read some books and listened to some podcasts that talk about how we need to reduce our footprint to 10 percent of what it currently is here in the United States. There are outrageous changes that can be made to get to that reduced number, and there are people who have made it to that benchmark. To them I say KUDOS!! But even if you can't get to 10 percent every little bit helps. While that 10 percent is a mighty fine goal, it might be too restrictive for you and that's okay because every little bit helps.

So, take that reusable bag to the store, but if you forget it in the car don't beat yourself up. If you want to go to the movies don't deny yourself the soda and popcorn because of the trash. You don't have to make every change, all at once. You just need to find what will work for you long term, something you can do every day. Have I said how every little bit helps? Well, it does and if you can't help at least don't do more harm.

It's not how low you can go; it's how long you can maintain it. Doing something for a week isn't going to break a bad habit...it takes being consistent for 60-90 days to make a real change. Unlike that fad diet you tried for 4 weeks and didn't see a change, or that new 30-day workout routine which built no muscles, to really change it has to be something you can sustain! Something that isn't so difficult that you can keep up and if at all possible, something that you are

passionate about or love. But most
importantly, it has to be
sustainable.

sus·tain·a·bil·i·ty

/səˌstānəˈbilədē/

noun

1. ***the ability to be maintained at a certain rate or level.***
   "the sustainability of economic growth"
2. avoidance of the depletion of natural resources in order to maintain an ecological balance.
   "the pursuit of global environmental sustainability"

Chapter Two

Why it matters

We all live on the same floating blue and green ball of dust in the same solar system, and until I'm told otherwise, the only planet in this system that can sustain life that is conducive to our body's needs.

Water

This wonderful world is 70% water, yet we can only drink about 2% of that water. We, ourselves, are made up of 60% water, and we need to drink water everyday if we want to live. You can go a week without food but only three days without water. Water is essential!!

Yet in this modern time of so many innovations and information at our fingertips there are millions of people who don't have access to clean water. From pollution to droughts there are several different reasons why they might not have water, so why are those of us with clean water so wasteful with something so precious. If we can only drink 2% of the water available, we really should be more concerned about how we use it and how we waste it.

The 2% fresh water we drink is the same water we flush down the toilet, wash our clothes, our bodies, our teeth, our dishes, and cook with. That 2% of fresh water is also, more importantly, used to irrigate our crops, water our lawns, fill our pools, and given to the livestock. That 2% of our drinking water is used to frack for oils, manufacture that new cell phone or car, and cool those nuclear fusion power plants. While I am not saying we should stop watering the animals or crops or stop taking showers, I am asking why we waste so much of it when we do them.

We hear on the news about this year's droughts being the worst on record, that is until next year of course. We can't continue to use the water as if it's never going to end. We will talk a little more about water usage in another chapter. I'm just pointing out things that we need to change...we'll talk about how later.

Air

Another aspect of this big blue ball is the atmosphere that separates our breathing layer from outer space, outer space being where the space station orbits; it's much thinner than you think. From the earth's crust to space, if we drove 55 miles per hour, it would take 1 hour, 7 minutes and 38 seconds to reach space. It takes less time to get to space than to get to work for some people!

All the air we breathe is in the first 7.5 miles of the atmosphere (the Troposphere)[2]. Yet we act like there are all these layers of atmosphere for

---

[2] Earth's Atmosphere: A Multi-layered Cake. NASA Global Climate Change. October 2019. https://climate.nasa.gov/news/2919/earths-atmosphere-a-multi-layered-cake

us to put pollution in; like a drop of food color will not be seen in the ocean but will be seen in a glass of water, we treat the atmosphere like it's that ocean when it's really an eight ounce glass. I, for one, want to breathe clean air, free of toxins that cause health issues.

Speaking of those toxins and pollutants, we drill and mine this planet for energy to heat and cool our homes, to fuel our cars and stoves, to make products that will never break down in nature in our lifetime and generally will only last us less than five years.

Energy

We blow the tops off of mountains and send the sludge sliding into the nearest river, stream or lake. We send people into those holes to mine for materials that took the planet eons to create, it takes us months to mine, and minutes to burn.

When that mine won't give any more we do it all again to another mountain top. Until we eventually run out of mountain tops and find some other way to get those fossil fuels. Speaking of....

We fracture the earth's surface to drill for natural gas in a shoal that doesn't want to give it up. We shoot liquids into those drilled holes we created at such a high pressure that makes little breaks in the ground underneath us that allow us to retrieve those fossil fuels that mother nature obviously never intended on us to have. That sequestered natural gas isn't without its carbon footprint. While it burns cleaner than those mountain top coal mines, the destruction it causes starts with those liquids that were pumped to fracture the earth. They can and have leaked into our groundwater (that 2% we can drink) and we don't even know what they are because they are company proprietary, and we wonder why our well is poisoned. Then to boot, shooting liquid into the earth and fracturing the surface causes earthquakes in areas where we don't have earthquake buildings codes and then wonder why the buildings are falling down and killing people.

Habitat Destruction

Speaking of killing, we are but one species on the planet; but we act like we are the only one that matters. There are 1.8 million <u>known</u> species on this planet[3], and millions more we probably don't know about (think of the ocean, we haven't explored all the depths of the ocean, so I am sure there are species we know nothing about...for now). So, what affects us also affects those other 1.7999 million species.

------

[3] National Geographic Resource Library. Biodiversity. Encyclopedia Enrty
https://education.nationalgeographic.org/resourc
e/biodiversity

We are killing off those species at a rate of between 200-2,000 a year which is 1,000 higher than the natural extinction rate[4], pre-industrial era. If we don't make changes to our behaviors, then it won't be too long before we are one of those 200-2000 species that just doesn't make it. We are destroying our own habitat, causing food and water shortages.

"Without environmental sustainability, economic stability and social cohesion cannot be achieved." By Phil Harding

---

[4] World Wildlife Foundation. Biodiversity. https://wwf.panda.org/discover/our_focus/biodiversity/biodiversity/

Chapter Three

Profit, People, Planet & Technology

"The first rule of sustainability is to align with natural forces, or at least not try to defy them."-Paul Hawken

Sustainability is measured over time and used to create changes, in ourselves, in our communities and in our country's rules and regulations. Sustainability has three pillars that must work together to create that change: the economy, the society, the environment or Profit, People, Planet.[5] However, in today's modern society, we have to also add technology into the equation. Let's take a look at each of the points that make up sustainability.

Economy (Profit). Each state, country, county, community, or city has to have ongoing resources necessary for their communities to meet their needs (not exceed their wants) for all businesses, and people involved.

---

[5] University of Alberta, Office of Sustainability. "What is Sustainability". https://www.mcgill.ca/sustainability/files/sustainability/what-is-sustainability.pdf

Example: City A has put solar arrays on the top of all buildings and homes in their city through federal and private energy grants. They have now created a regulation in the building code that all new buildings or homes must have solar arrays on the roofs moving forward. This is sustainable because the cost of solar panels has reduced significantly over the years making it economical for the construction businesses to be able to add that to the other building requirements in the city.

This also works with family budget ideas too. The economy of the family. If you have more money going out than coming in, it's not sustainable. You have to figure out how to reduce your expenses and/or increase your income. We always start with what we can cut back on. Do we really need eight streaming programs when we only actually use three?

Society (People). Upholding the values that create fairness and equality for all people in the community, regardless of homogeneous status.

> Example: The Christian, Satanist, and Muslim religions are all able to have gathering places at the same cost per square foot with no restrictions on where they can build or buy.

Any change we want to make has to be in line with our values, if we want to be able to continue it for any length of time. If we aren't true to who we are then any change we make is only for the benefit of others and will eat away at us until we can no longer keep the facade up or we lose ourselves. Much like taking a job we don't love, we resent having to get up every morning to go there because we don't love it, we don't even like it. If you have a job you love or are passionate about, your job isn't really a job but a calling or a purpose. However, you have to find what you are passionate about to find that calling.

How do you find what you are passionate about? That passion lives inside of you. What do you value? What do you believe in? What do you look forward to doing? What would you do if money was not an issue? Inside you lies the answers to those questions, and those answers will help show you what you love and in turn what you are passionate about.

Me? I am passionate about the environment that I live in. I value having clean drinking water. I love being able to ride my paddleboard without seeing trash on the water (which I pick up and place in a bag for disposal on shore). I enjoy being able to scuba dive and only see fish, not bottles. I value being able to breathe fresh air that doesn't smell like some kind of mineral. However, most importantly, I value my children and I want them to have the same forest, lakes, and rivers to swim in, I want their children's children to have that chance too. To do that, my passion lies in helping others understand the importance of making changes to reduce their carbon footprint.

Environment (Planet). Ensuring that the natural resources are used at a rate in which the planet can replenish themselves for continued use.

We fight in wars over just a handful of things; ideologies (cultures), religions, and natural resources. We fight over natural resources because we know that they aren't infinite, that some resources take eons to replace (think coal and natural gas) and we know they are valuable to our way of life (A/C in the summer and heat in the winter) and we want to make sure that we have them for ourselves and our families. We wouldn't feel the need to have to fight for them if everyone was living within their needs....not their wants. What we are doing to the planet, our demands on the planet and the resources **Isn't Sustainable**!

We have a habit of using more resources than the planet can replenish. We live as though all we want is available all the time. That just isn't true, and every year it gets worse with the increase in global population and climate change. In 2006, when the first overshoot day was determined, we overshot the ability of the planet to replenish the natural resources used by August 21st. We can go backwards in time and see that in 1971 (the year after the first Earth Day) we hit that date on December 25th. As you can see, every year that day moves forward. In 2021 that date was July 29th[6]. The overshoot day is determined by the formula:

(Earth's Biocapacity / Humanity's Ecological Footprint) x 365 = Earth Overshoot Day

In my lifetime we have never not overused the natural resources available, and we continue to overshoot the Earth every year.

Overshooting the natural resources is the equivalent of running out of money in the middle of the month with no more money coming in

---

[6] About Earth Overshoot Day.
https://www.overshootday.org/about-earth-overshoot-day/

until the first. It isn't sustainable. I know I use that word a lot but if you can't keep it going it doesn't help in the long run.

For something to be sustainable it has to fulfill all three pillars for there to be balance in sustainability.

In addition to the three pillars, for an environmental policy to be created technology has to be included. We come into the idea of changing the world and protecting the planet all bright eyed and bushy tailed but there is so much more than "it's good for the environment" to take into consideration for something to change. That is why the fourth pillar of sustainability is Technology.

Technology is ever changing and upgrading. As it does, it allows for things that were just a pipe dream 10 years ago to be the new normal. Basically, normal is relative and ever changing. An example is solar panels. They were uber expensive in the 1980s costing more than 100 times what they cost today and they were harder to find. Now you can go to any sporting goods store and buy a pocket solar array to charge your phone while camping for $30.

Landfills have learned through technology how to capture that methane gas that is created through the decomposition of our waste. They have learned how to turn that captured methane into energy to power homes instead of burning the gas or allowing it to just leak into the atmosphere.

What we have to keep in mind is that any changes we need to or want to make, don't disadvantage one section of the population over another. That they aren't so expensive as to put undue financial pressure on the population. That there is actual tangible technology that will allow for the change to be made, and that in the end we can't cause more harm to the planet than before.

*"Earth provides enough to satisfy every man's needs, but not every man's greed." —
Mahatma Gandhi*

Chapter Four

Where to start

The hardest part of starting a new routine or challenge is that first step. Where to start, how to start; the important thing to remember is just to start! Everyone's starting point is going to be different based on what they have already done and what they already know. It doesn't matter if you are a hundred steps behind or in front of your friends, so long as we are all on the same journey.

Start with a checklist to take inventory, grab a notebook and pen.

1. Call up or check the website for your recycling and solid waste hauler to see what is and is not acceptable recycling.
2. Take a look in your recycling bin. Did you "wish-cycle" anything?

"Wish cycling" is wanting something to be recyclable and

placing it in your curbside recycling bin hoping that your recycling hauler will be able to recycle it or figure out how to recycle it for you. There are places you can go to figure out where something is able to be recycled or if it's recyclable at all. A good website for that is Earth911.com.

> 3. Take a look in your trash bin. Are there any accepted recycling materials in the trash bin?

Now that the basics are done, let's move on to making a mindset change. When it comes to mindset changes, we first have to know where our mind is set. To do this we have to practice mindfulness.

Mindfulness means to be in the moment, in the present, to pay attention to things that we usually autopilot...life. Mindfulness is paying attention to our body, to our thoughts, to our feelings, to our surroundings and then, without judgment, finding what makes us better people. Mindfulness is all the rage right now. Everyone knows the buzz word, but do they understand the meaning?

"Mindfulness is deliberately paying full attention to what is happening around you— in your body, heart, and mind. Mindfulness is awareness without criticism or judgment." – Jan Chozen Bays

Sitting with and paying attention to ourselves is the key to mindfulness. Next, it's helpful to write down the things we do. We have a habit of making a "to do list" of things we HAVE to get done, so let's start by making a habits list. Once we have taken the time to sit with ourselves and pay attention to what we do on a regular basis, determine which of those things we are doing we can or want to change.

Then we can make a "goals" list of the things we want to change. As we try the changes, mark the item off making our "ta done list" to see what we do and how we do it. Make notes next to things that don't work with a simple explanation as to why it didn't work. That way we can go back later on and see if we can tweak the item and try again.

When going to restaurants, be mindful of your drink order and remember to say "no thank you" to the straw so long as you don't have a medical condition that requires you to use a straw...then use the straw.

If you usually take a doggy bag home with you for what you haven't finished at the restaurant, then before you head out, grab a storage container and put it in your purse or bag so you don't need to ask for that "to-go box". This will reduce food waste because you are taking the extra food, from that super-size portion, home for lunch tomorrow. You are also reducing trash waste by not having a takeout container to throw away later. Best of all, you are reducing wasting your time. Taking that container with you allows you to skip a step once you get the food home. Since the majority of to-go containers are foam, which you shouldn't use to reheat in the microwave, you'd have to remove it from the to-go container and place in a microwave safe container. Now instead of having to do any of that, the container you took with you to the restaurant will be able to go from the fridge to the microwave to the dishwasher without issue. No waste, no fuss.

We have all heard the "don't go to the grocery store hungry" or "don't go to the store without a list" sayings, they are said for a reason. We mindlessly wander the aisles and find ourselves buying more food than we need or can use before it goes bad, which leads to food waste. And food waste leads to wasting our hard-earned money.

Impulse shopping is another reason to have a list with you. As you stand there in line waiting for the elderly lady in the front to finish writing a check, you glance around at the little bags of chips, candy bars, charging cable...and think to yourself, "I am a little hungry from all this shopping" or "I think I remember someone saying they needed a new charging cable" and you grab an item you don't really need at all because you mindlessly saw it and your brain was like "sure, why not". This is in the same realm as mindful eating.

Don't just sit on the couch Netflixing with a bag of chips. Next thing you'll know the bag of chips is gone and you have no recollection of eating them. Be in the moment with your eating, with your driving, and with your shopping. While you are in that moment look at the packaging that the items come in. Here is the third part of shopping...packaging.

Another spot where we can be mindful of our environment is in the types of packaging our items come in. There is no universal recycling guide, each municipal or recycling hauler across the country collects and sorts what materials their Material Recovery Facility (MRF) is set up for and which materials manufacturers in their area are accepting.

In Washington State they can recycle those orange juice and milk cartons, but in Nevada they can't.

In California they have organics recycling (food waste and yard debris) in Florida they do not.

It's important to take a few moments to call or check the website for your recycling haulers to see what you can recycle in your curbside recycling and THEN use that information, not only to make sure you aren't wish-cycling, but that when you need to buy items, you buy items that have packaging that can be recycled in your curbside cart or in your local area.

Even better would be to go second hand! Thrift stores, friends, and rentals. An example is Home Depot, if you need to remove some tile flooring and it isn't your job, you can rent a hammer drill for a day or a week for less than the cost of the tool and you don't have to worry about space in the garage or shed for it after the task is done. There is no need to become your own hardware store if you only need the tool for one project.

"How we pay attention to the present moment largely determines the character of our experience, and therefore, the quality of our lives." –
Sam Harris

Chapter Five

The 7 R's

Seven!? What happened to the simple "Reduce, reuse, recycle" we all grew up on? Where did all these extra Rs come from? What do they mean? And are they as important as those first three Rs we all know and love.

The first thing to ask is where in the world did these little chasing arrows come from and how did they come to mean Reduce, Reuse and Recycle. Those chasing arrows can be seen everywhere now. They are on the notebooks we write in, the plastics our things come in, the plastic bag we put those items in. The problem is that in an attempt to be more sustainable we have weaved the past in with the present with our eye on the future.

The recycling symbol, as we know it, has only been around since the first Earth Day in April 1970. Gary Anderson, a UCLA student entered a contest, held by the Container

Corporation of America, to create a symbol for this new environmental campaign and he won! Because of the popularity of Earth Day and the environmental campaigns that have come since, we have used that symbol to mean recycling. Now here is the kicker...those chasing arrows "Reduce, Reuse, Recycle" doesn't actually mean that something is recyclable.

Depending on the material the symbol on it could mean that it's made from recycled materials. Think about your paper towels or bathroom tissue, they have a symbol on their packaging, but those paper products are at the end of their life cycle and unable to be recycled anywhere! That symbol on their packaging is signaling that they are Made from recycled materials (Post-consumer).

There are no government regulations on how to use the symbol. Therefore, on plastics, the industry puts the resin number (plastic type) inside the recycling symbol for the Material Recovery Facilities (MRF) to know what type of polymer it is so they can sort them into the correct lines. That little number lets the manufactures, that are using recyclable materials, know at what temperature the products will melt to create something new.

There isn't a symbol on glass or metal, but they are two materials that can be recycled indefinitely without losing their integrity. Both paper and plastics can only be recycled a certain number of times before the fibers or polymer chains are too small to hold. I want you to know that we aren't going to recycle our way out of climate change, but as I have said repeatedly, every little bit helps. Okay... back to the Rs.

****

The 7 R's: Rethink/Refuse, Reduce, Reuse, Repurpose, Repair, Recycle, and Rot! It isn't the process of just one item but something to do with every item at different steps in its consumer life cycle. When we think about our stuff we need to keep in mind from the creation of the item to the end of its life.

The first step is to **RETHINK/REFUSE** . This doesn't mean to deny what you need, just to think about what you truly need or want. When family members start to give things away, do you really need to take that second dining room table and chairs that were once in Aunt Helen's house? If you do want it, can you sell your current dining room set to make room for it? Just don't take it and sit it in storage. If you don't want it and it's in good shape take it to Goodwill, put it on Facebook Marketplace, make some money on it or give it away for free. Either use it or <u>refuse it</u>!!

Here's another example without a sentimental hold, I love going to the thrift store and garage sales, but to make sure that I am only buying what I need, if I see something I really like and I have another like it, I have to be able to part with the one I have....I don't need two of them!

Now when you go to the store, you use a basket or cart to pick out and carry your items around the store. When you get to the counter, <u>REFUSE</u> a bag (paper or plastic). Scan the items and put them back in the basket or cart and just place them in your car or truck or backpack, or maybe those reusable bags you accidentally left in the car, instead of using a single use bag.

"But wait a minute! I use those bags more than once, I use them in my wastebaskets, or to clean up after my pets. What am I to do if I refuse them? Now I have to spend more of my hard-earned money to buy small poop bags or wastebasket bags." That's hard-earned money you could be spending on other things you need and that is a valid point! I'm not going to tell you not to do it then, but I am going to ask the hard question...Do you have a large bag of bags in your pantry, under the sink, in a closet?? Could you REFUSE a single use bag <u>every other time </u>you go to the store or, and hear me out, you could use the bread bag, dry cleaners bag or the bread bag to clean up the pet poo or as a liner for your wastebasket...all of which are bags you already bought other things in that would otherwise go in the trash can empty and on to the landfill or waste to energy plant. At least this way you can reuse them to hold other waste.

We are looking for low not zero.

Next up is **REDUCE**. Reduce the amount of a product you use. Use a pea size amount of toothpaste instead of that swoop the advertisements show or a nickel size amount of shampoo instead of a palm size. Reduce the number of those single use bags from the store (see refuse) you bring home. I'm sure your bread won't mind sharing space in the reusable bag with your chips or even the eggs. Instead of using those produce bags, let the fruit and veggies breathe loosely or if you feel you need them to be contained in a bag, try one of those reusable net produce bags...or that net bag from the onions or oranges you bought last week.

Do you really need a single use water bottle? Can you buy a stainless steel water bottle that you can reuse all day long and again tomorrow? You can't reuse those single use plastic bottles a second day and here is why: it's the same reason you shouldn't leave those plastic bottles of water in a hot car. When those single use plastic bottles are heated, in the hot car or in the sink to kill the bacteria in them from yesterday's use, it releases chemicals into your water. So, you can't clean and reuse a single-use plastic bottle, and you can't not clean out your backwash and bacteria from using it yesterday. Now, if you don't want to buy one of those stainless steel or glass water bottles then you can use the old spaghetti sauce jar or a mason jar as your travel water bottle.

Let's take a look at the bathroom...instead of taking a 30-minute shower or a bath, take a 5–10-minute shower. When it's time to replace your toilet, replace it with a low flow; until then put a brick in the tank to displace the water, it will still flush! Make sure to turn the water OFF while you brush your teeth. That bath towel you use to dry off, after your 8-minute shower, can be used for up to (but not more than) three times before it needs to be washed.

If you aren't using an electric item, unplug it so it doesn't siphon energy from the outlet, no need to pay for something you aren't actually using at this moment.

Instead of buying another shirt or pants, check your closet and drawers. Are there clothes you haven't worn in a while? Why haven't you worn them? Do they not fit, out of style, not your style anymore? Maybe you find that pair of jeans that somehow got pushed all the way to the back that you absolutely love! Kudos for finding them again!! But if you look and all you see is that there is a trash bag worth of clothes that you don't want or need...send them to the thrift store not the landfill. In most locations textiles are not recyclable in your curbside bin. Now take a few weeks to see if you need to replace any of those clothes. If you do need to replace any of those clothes from the bag of clothes, start with the local thrift store instead of the mall. Buying second hand helps continue the demand for reused items, there is no packaging, AND, in most places, no sales tax.

Change what you do have to buy by finding reusable alternatives. Instead of paper towels use cloth towels that you can wash and reuse! Instead of dryer sheets, use wool balls with a few drops of essential oils. A lot of these sound familiar, and they are because they were what we did before we turned our economy into a disposable one.

We are looking for low not zero.

#3 **REUSE.** This means using the item for the exact purpose that it was created for. The bread bag used to clean up fido's poop is a form of reusing. A bag is a bag is a bag. Reuse the jar that the pickles came in to hold your homemade kimchi... a jar is a jar is a jar. Reuse isn't a sexy R but it's a good one.

We are looking for low not zero.

The next one is **REPURPOSE**. Now this one is a bit more fun. Remember that jar that was reused to hold your homemade kimchi? Well now it's going to hold screws in the garage because there's a chip in the treads and the lid doesn't work. The old t-shirt from the closet clean out that has holes in it or was too stained to go to the thrift store...is now a set of those reusable towels. Or do a little cutting and tying and you can make yourself some produce bags!

Repurposing, unlike reusing, is taking something and giving it a new life as something else. A lot of the time the items we send to the recycling center are repurposed. A plastic water bottle doesn't always become a water bottle again, sometimes its new life is decking, carpet, or the fluff in a winter coat. Those single use plastic bags, when they can't be recycled again into more plastic bags, become a park bench or birdhouse. It was "recycled" and made into something that has less value, it has been downcycled. The reason we call it that is because changing it to a park bench or carpet has ended its chance to be reused or repurposed and unable to be recycled again. If we take something and give it a new life that is better than what it was AND it still remains recyclable, it's called upcycling. Like taking those soda tabs and turning them into a chain for your purse is an example of upcycling. The chain has more value than those tabs alone and whenever you want to change out the "chain" those tabs are still recyclable.

**We are looking for low
not zero.**

R number five is pretty self-explanatory...**REPAIR**. Now we can't repair everything but we can repair a lot. Instead of buying a new cell phone when the screen breaks, repair it. Instead of buying a new pair of shoes when the sole starts coming apart, repair it. Heels that broke, repair it. Zipper that isn't working on that jacket you like, repair it. Lawn mower blades dull, sharpen them instead of buying new ones. You get the idea, right?

**We are looking for low
not zero.**

Six is the well-known **RECYCLE**. But you have to be careful with this one as every municipality is different based on the haulers and Material Recovery Facility (MRF) they use. Some MRFs only do cardboard. Oh, and that cereal box you have, it isn't cardboard...its backer board or chipboard. It's considered mixed paper. If the cardboard doesn't have the zigzag pattern on the inside, it's actually paper.

Paper needs to be clean of food or oils AND flat. I know if you are like I used to be, I used to ball up the paper after I had finished with it. But the machinery that sorts paper actually needs it flat, so it doesn't get mistaken for a 3D item (containers). So, flatten out those balls of paper and they typically need to be at least the size of a credit card (business cards are too small as are the tags from clothes). If you have books you want to recycle, you'll need to pull the hardcover off. Notebooks need to have the metal spiral removed. If you shred your paper, put it in a paper bag not a cardboard box or a plastic bag. Speaking of plastic....

Not all plastics are taken at every MRF, it depends on if there is a market for the item. Not all plastics have value. For a plastic to have value there has to be some kind of market demand for it. If the composition of the plastic makes it too expensive to melt, repair and reuse, there is no market...no market translates into not collected, not sorted, not sellable. Most places will take the PET #1, soda and water bottles. PET #1 is a shiny plastic that is easy to crush. Number #2s are usually taken too...those are the milk jugs and detergent bottles. You can find the number of the plastics inside those chasing arrows recycling symbols...which doesn't mean it's recyclable just that it "could be recyclable" or that it's made from recycled materials.

On to metal, that tuna can is recyclable, but your frying pan might not be accepted in your curbside or apartment complex recycling cart/bin/container because it isn't accepted at the MRF. Some metals have to go to a scrap metal yard not your curbside recycling bin. A general rule on metals is if your food or drink CAME in it (as well as your pets), it's probably accepted. Soup/ Fruit/ Veggie/ Pets' food cans, tuna/ spam/ crab/ cat food tins, pie tins, and aluminum foil. The pie tin and foil will need to be clean of food or grease and balled up to the size of your fist. You can save all the larger metal items and take them to a scrap metal yard and sell them for money or you can find a recycling drop off location and dispose of them there, just not in the commingled bins.

Glass is another one that's tricky. Most MRFs (if they accept glass) only accept bottles and jars. Wine, beer, some non-alcoholic drink bottles or pickle jars, etc.; NO bakeware, cookware, dinnerware. The reason for this is that the latter is treated to withstand higher temperatures than the former, so they melt at different rates. That's not helpful for the manufacturer to reuse. They need all the glass to melt at the same rate. There could also be a color requirement for your glass. Some MRFs only accept clear, green or brown. It's all they have a market for. So if you think they won't notice that really pretty purple vase, they will...and it could mess up the end product costing the manufacturer more money and mistrust of recyclable materials...then we lose recycling all together.

Side note on recycling: Keep America Beautiful (KAB) was created by the manufacturers (Coca-Cola and Pepsi) whose products can be recycled. It was created to take the ownership of the cradle-to-cradle responsibility of the item off them and put it on the consumer.

The bottle bills in most states went the way of the dodo when KAB was created. That way the manufacturers didn't have to worry about what was happening to their product, how it was used or disposed of and didn't have to worry about making sure that some locations deposit fees were paid. The litter bugs were us and WE could all fix the problem with recycling. We aren't going to recycle our way out of climate change. That's why recycling is the sixth R and not the first R.

One more thing about plastics. Plastic wrap, plastic film, flexible plastics, or plastic bags are all a NO-NO in your curbside recycling. The only place those can be recycled is at locations that recycle nothing else in that bin but them. Plastic films (film, wrap, bags) all tangle up the MRF machinery and cause it to have to stop running. When the machinery has to shut down for cleaning, an actual person is going to need to go into that part of the MRF and hand clean all that film off the machinery so it can continue to run and sort. So don't be that guy...don't put your recyclable materials into a plastic bag in your recycling bin. Take that film back to the local retailer and recycle it in the specialty bin in their lobby area. If you are concerned about the cleanliness of your recycling bin then put a large bag in your bin to hold the recyclable materials but make sure that the bag won't come loose when the container is dumped and when it needs to be changed out; use it for your trash so it doesn't go to the landfill without a good use.

We are looking for low not zero.

Last, but not least, is **ROT**. Like repair, not everything can rot, but those items that can, should. In the United States, we use a tremendous amount of land, energy, and water for food production. The biggest land user is of course animals...I'm not saying run out there and be a vegan, but I am asking that if you buy a steak, you use it before it goes bad, don't throw it out.

Big energy and water users are our vegetables, grains, and fruits. Here is the sad truth about them: 25 percent of all food grown is left in the field, on the vine or in the trees because it isn't "pretty enough". The USDA actually had on the books how food was supposed to look. An apple had to be a certain shape, if it grew with a nose on it...it was left on the tree to eventually fall off, why waste money on paying folks to pick fruit that can't be sold because it's ugly. If the zucchini was too big or too small, it was left on the vine.

We have food insecurity all across the world, and here we are leaving food to rot on the vine because it isn't pretty enough...it doesn't look like all the other apples in the bunch. You know who doesn't care what they look like? Food!!!

Now you are probably thinking, isn't this the ROT section and isn't that food in fact rotting? And the answer to both is yes. But what I am getting to is that 25 percent of all food grown is wasted before it even makes it to the trucks and grocery stores. And so is the energy, water and land used to grow it.

On top of that 25 percent wasted, it is estimated that 40 percent of food bought is landfilled. Are you kidding me!!!! We have stores throwing out food two days before expiration date and locking their dumpsters so no one can forage for perfectly good food. Why are they throwing it out? BECAUSE no one wants to buy food whose expiration date is too short for them to get it home and use it. The crazy thing is those expiration dates mean little.

The food industry started those dates so that you'd use it and buy some more and do it often. There is no standard for expiration dates on any food with the exception of baby formula. Take a stroll through the grocery store, you'll see "sell by", "use by", "best by", they can make up any date they want, the government doesn't care, and the industry isn't going to regulate themselves. That's the wolf watching the hen house! Those dates tell you when the item has reached peak flavor, or freshness but it doesn't go bad that very day. It depends on how you store the item when you get it home.

"We won't have a society if we destroy the environment." –
Margaret Mead

What is the takeaway I'm trying to get to? All I am asking is for you to think about going to the local farmers market and asking for that ugly fruit! When you do go to the grocery store instead of buying a bag of oranges, if you generally throw at least one or two away, pick out your oranges individually. Don't buy more than you can use in the time frame that they will go bad. But when they do go bad...compost them, don't landfill them! You can live in a house, a farm, or an apartment and still compost. You can have a big 3'x3' compost bin or a 10-gallon Rubbermaid tote full of worms. If you learn the carbon to nitrogen ratio there won't be much of a smell and the soil that is made will make all the flowers, or whatever you grow, very happy. If you are lucky enough to be in an area that does organic recycling, make sure to opt into the program.

The Seven Rs can save you
green as well as help "save the planet".

"Composting is the natural process of recycling organic matter, such as leaves and food scraps, into a valuable fertilizer that can enrich soil and plants." - NPR, July 2020

Chapter Six

Composting

Just my two cents—Composting doesn't have to be just for your food, think bio pods instead of a coffin that doesn't break down quickly. Become a Tree, and live forever.

Not all food can be composted

in a backyard composter, but every little bit helps. There is food waste from the fields to your garbage bin. Even if you wanted to go zero waste on this one, without a municipal composting program you are going to be left with some waste that wouldn't be able to be composted. So don't beat yourself up on the inability to be zero food waste. Since you are being more careful about the amount you buy so you can use it before it goes bad, there are still some things you don't eat and become waste; the core of an apple, the peel of a banana, the ends of a scallion.

Not all composters are the same in what they can take and how they work, but one thing is the same in all the different styles of composter...the necessary ratio of Carbon to Nitrogen. The C:N ratio is 25 to 1. Too much carbon and it will take FOREVER for your food scraps to decompose. On the flip side, too much nitrogen and you'll have that stinky pile no one wants to be around. It may sound a bit difficult but you'll get the hang of it pretty quickly.

There are several different types of bins that we will talk about from the small worm bin (vermicomposting) to your large backyard "pitchfork and turn" bin and a little something in between.

Let's begin with an easy to maintain worm bin that can fit into any house/apartment size and the amount of worms needed is all dependent on the amount of food scraps you have. Since we are reducing our waste and refusing what we don't need, we might not need too many worms!

Now you can DIY or buy a bin. There are plenty of YouTube videos showing how to make a worm bin and plenty of sites out there willing to sell you one. After you build or buy the bin you'll need to get the home ready for your wiggly friends. You'll need some shredded, damp paper or cardboard for the bedding of the worms and for a cover layer and food scraps. Remember the Carbon to Nitrogen ratio here to make sure your worms can do what they need to do. Now their bin is ready to be their home, you'll need some creepy crawlers to eat those food scraps. The best and most effective vermicomposting worms are the Red Wigglers. For every pound of worms, two pounds of food scraps.

If you decide to go the DIY route, you can make these bins from five-gallon buckets, Rubbermaid totes, stackable garden nursery flats...you are only limited by your imagination on how to create the bin. You just need to make sure there is enough space for your worms to migrate away from heat and humidity and towards food.

Now, there are a few things to remember with the worms, they don't like citrus or it getting too hot! The worms will migrate to where the food is and leave behind amazing compost for potted plants (outside) and gardens. That black gold composting isn't the only thing they leave behind. A byproduct of vermicomposting is a juice I like to call "worm tea". You'll need some way of capturing that juice to use on your vegetable garden but really, you'll want to have a drain hole so that the juice doesn't just collect in the bottom of the bin making the soil too wet. If it's too wet, it creates humidity and heat for those red wigglers, plus if the juice is still in there the composting will be too wet to get out.

The worm tea is a great plant food while the plants are growing, but use on outside plants only, as there could be some tiny insects that are attracted to the tea and beat you there. No one wants little flying bugs in their house.

The worms can make it over the winter and summer so long as you feed them and don't let them get too cold (below 40 degrees Fahrenheit) or too hot (over 80 degrees Fahrenheit). They will reproduce so you'll need to start a second bin or give some of them away to someone else who wants to start a worm bin. Sharing is caring and sharing your worms and your knowledge is priceless.

If you want a more "traditional" composting bin, then you are probably thinking of the tumbler...it doesn't have little wigglers to freak you out or worry you about accidentally killing them from the heat or cold. You can buy one or make one...the size and design are up to you.

The tumbler is just what it sounds like. The tumbler is a barrel with small holes to allow for air to aerate the mixture to help with decomposition. Again, you must make sure that your carbon to nitrogen ratio is correct so there isn't any odor, and it has what it needs to break down to make perfectly good composting.

Simply put in your food scraps, some moist cardboard or paper and give it a good couple of turns. Then every day you'll want to go out and give it a turn to make sure that there is oxygen in there to help break down the food waste. If it starts to smell...there could be too much moisture, or the ratio is off.

If you have a big space and really want to go all out and have a big composting pile to take care of yours and maybe the neighbors food scraps, you can make a large pitch-and-turn composting pile; there are two types. The first is the two or three bin piles where you start the pile in one bin and when it's time to turn it, you pitchfork it into the other bin, adding more carbon and nitrogen to keep feeding the bin. Or the one bin where you remove the barrel or wiring around the compost and pitchfork the decomposing mixture back into the bin in a new location. Now, once the temperature reaches 160 degrees Fahrenheit, you'll want to stop turning the bin to keep it cooking. You'll know when it's done when the temperature starts to decrease.

The second is a dump and go style. Here you make a pile and just keep dumping nitrogen (organics) and carbon (cardboard or paper) with the occasional turn. But really just letting mother nature do her thing. Or if you have chickens...let them do the aerating for you. They are awesome little compost makers, plus their bedding is nitrogen rich.

So, we talked about the worms, the tumbler, the pitchfork and the dump and go. One more way to compost goes hand in hand with gardening. If you don't garden, you can do any of the other composting options but if you do garden…lasagna gardening is cool!

Lasagna gardening is at the end of the growing cycle when you are getting ready to winterize your garden for next year. What you will do is use food scraps and cardboard and/or yard debris, you'll layer the food scraps and cardboard in the garden bed. Make sure to get it good and high so it can break down all winter long keeping the ground warm while creating compost right there on the site where it will be needed in the spring. Cover the top of the lasagna layering with a final layer of straw to keep the birds from picking through your garden lasagna for food scraps.

Now I do have an interesting bit of information about those awesome green compostable single use bags.... they aren't compostable in your backyard composter. They only break down in a commercial or industrial compost pile. Your backyard composter will not get hot enough to break those bags down. AND because they are compostable, they are NOT recyclable. If your municipality doesn't compost, those bags are not worth your time or money for food scraps. You can use them in place of trash bags, but not in your composting bins.

Composting is a fantastic way to use those food scraps, but it's also a great way to fertilize fields which can really help the environment. Composting on a large scale could actually help with those red algae blooms and dead zones in the oceans. How, you ask? With the reduction of chemical runoff from farms, vineyards, orchards, etc.

Everything we do costs money. Growing veggies costs money. Raising livestock costs money. We need to make enough to continue to do the thing and make enough to buy the stuff we need.

Let's give an example, these numbers and figures can vary depending on region and supply and demand, but they will suffice for the purposes of our example, let's take a look at a loaf of bread.

The wheat farmer spends .05 cents to grow a bushel, he's going to want to make .07 cents for that same bushel...cost plus labor. The baker, who buys the bushel at .07 cents, is going to add that 7 cents to the cost of all the other ingredients to make that loaf of bread...the baker's total cost is .75 cents per loaf. He's going to want to charge the grocery store that orders it $1.00. The store is going to charge us $1.50.

If that farmer wants to make more money, he has two ways of doing it: increase his asking price (which most farmers can't do because the cost is determined by the federal government and subsidized by that same government) or get more customers. To get more customers he has to grow more. If he can't increase his farm size, the next best thing is to figure out how to grow bigger, fuller crops of wheat on the land he has. Now he isn't increasing his "carbon footprint" by land size, but he does based on how he increases his crop yield.

In comes pesticides, herbicides, and fertilizer. Now if that farmer is composting then he can use that composting to fertilize his land. He could also do a crop rotation. He's probably going to also use some pesticide or herbicide to help keep the bugs off the crop. If that farmer isn't composting enough for his crop size he's going to use bag fertilizer. Those bagged fertilizers have a high level of nitrogen and phosphorus in them to help the crop grow faster and fuller. But they also do the same for the weeds too...so then there are more pesticides or herbicides which take the nutrients out of the ground causing the farmer to need more bagged fertilizer and then the rain.

The rain will wash away into the ditches any of the pesticides, herbicides or fertilizer that is sitting on the topsoil. Water looks for the path of least resistance, and flows to the nearest river, stream, creek, lake, etc. Which will find its way to the ocean. That increased phosphorus and nitrogen is what causes the red algae blooms, those blooms are causing a drop in oxygenation in the water that kills the fish causing dead zones.

The farmer has fuller crops of wheat and got himself more customers, but the shrimper or fisherman is now struggling...not sustainable. Moral of the story: use natural compost or manure and your crops will require less chemicals and you don't kill off another industry.

For a list of items that are compostable from around the house, check out the list at the end of this book.

Chapter Seven

Water Usage

"Plans to protect air and water, wilderness and wildlife are in fact plans to protect man." – Stewart Udal

We learned earlier that

there is a lot of water on this

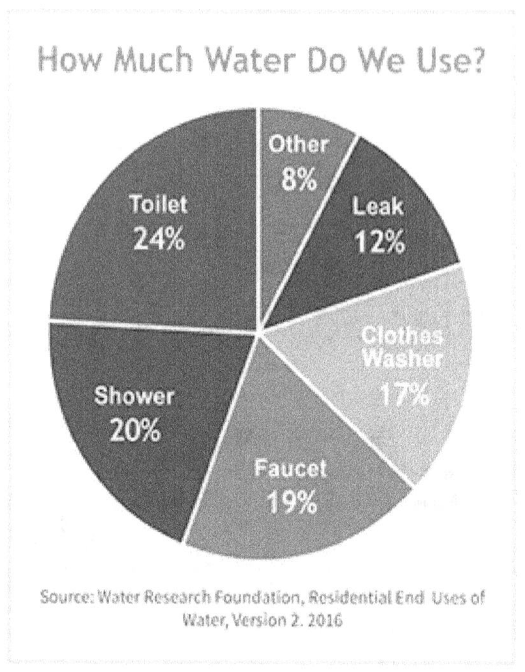

Source: Water Research Foundation, Residential End Uses of Water, Version 2. 2016

planet but only about 2% of that
water is drinkable (freshwater).
With the increase of droughts, that
2% feels like one. We have to
figure out ways to reduce what we
use, not only on a personal level,
but on a large scale- government
private company scale.

The Environmental
Protection Agency reports that

30% of the average American's water usage annual is OUTSIDE. Watering lawns, trees, gardens, and washing cars. The other 70% is indoors. The breakdown looks like this:

12% on leaks!! What a waste!

The average American uses approximately 80 gallons a day. We can find ways to reduce that number easily. The low hanging fruit is to start with those leaks! If there is a leak somewhere make sure to fix it ASAP. This not only saves water but depending on where the leak is could save you on having to redo walls, ceilings, floors, subfloors, foundations (if it goes long enough).

Next lowest fruit is to reduce your shower time. It is estimated that for each minute you are in the shower you are using 2 gallons of water. So, stop taking that 20 minute shower and instead opt for an 8 minute shower. Can you imagine the water used for a bath? I think that last time I had to fill the tub it took somewhere around 30 minutes to fill...or 60 gallons of water.

Next is to turn off the water while you brush your teeth or shave your face/legs. Since we brush our teeth for two minutes there's no reason to waste that four gallons of water.

Here is another easy one...don't run the dishwasher until it's full or run a load of laundry until it's full. As for rinsing dishes and recyclables, fill a bucket or basin with water, less than a half-gallon will work for rinsing both dishes and recyclables. Or better yet, when you go to rinse the fruits and vegetables off for dinner, rinse them over that bucket/basin so you capture the water then use it to rinse the dishes and recyclables after dinner. Easy peasy!

Reducing that toilet usage would require that "if it's yellow, let it mellow" saying. But you can't do that more than maybe a few pees before it starts to smell. So, that is one that's on you to decide. I will confess, I can't really do that one because the smell is too much for me. So, I take a 5-minute shower except on hair washing days when I use that extra three minutes.

We have taken a look at the inside, so on to the outside. Reduce your usage of water on the lawn and ornamental landscaping by changing them to native plants. Native plants will be able to survive on the water that is dropping from the sky and not contingent on you for water. If you garden, then make sure to water in the evening or early morning to reduce the amount of evaporation that will happen before the soil can absorb that water. Whenever possible, use drip irrigation instead of a sprinkler system. With the drip irrigation it waters the plant near the root to reduce evaporation and allows you to water less often and for less time.

Government-private companies also need to reduce their water usage but the only way that you can have a hand in that is with your votes and your dollar. We will talk about that in a little while.

I just want to say that there has been some innovation in the last decade in the use of greywater systems and recycling water at some of the industries out there. And in the systems, you can put in your home.

If you own your home, you can look into greywater systems to help irrigate plants in your yard so long as they aren't fruit bearing. So, shade trees and grass.

What is a greywater system you may ask? Greywater is water that you have already used in the house in some way that didn't come in contact with fecal matter. So, like the shower, the laundry, and sinks. The greywater system then redirects those "sewage" lines to a filtration system attached to your irrigation system that you can use, like I said on trees and grass. It's not dirty water, it's just got a gray tint to it. Now you might have to change up some of your cleaning supplies to use a greywater system to make sure they aren't harmful to the vegetation. The greywater system is a great way to capture some more of those 80 gallons a day you use. It's estimated that you could save somewhere in the neighborhood of 50-80% of your household wastewater by using a greywater system.

So, we have figured out some simple ways to reduce our water usage, and now we have talked about ways to reuse the water we do need to use!

Chapter Eight

Don't beat yourself up

New Year's resolutions are the worst thing we do to ourselves. We generally keep them for maybe a few weeks. Or we'll start our new diets next Monday (worse day to start a new habit, Wednesday is a much better day to start) and we might be able to do it for a few more weeks than those resolutions; but at some point we fall off the wagon and what do we do? We beat ourselves up for failing and then quit.

That's completely unnecessary. Success without failures doesn't happen! Two steps forward, one step back isn't going to kill anyone. There are going to be setbacks, there are going to be cheat days, there are going to be obstacles to stumble over before you are able to maneuver around them. That's life! Nothing worth having is easy, and anything too easy probably isn't worth having.

There will be days you forget those reusable bags. There might be days that takeout food is the only real option. There will be days when you forget your reusable water bottle, or you are out so long that you have to get a single use one because no place you visit has a refill station. All or any of these things happening doesn't mean you failed, it doesn't mean that you need to give up because "obviously it's too hard". It just means you had a stumble, a hiccup, a moment of pause. Now pick yourself up, brush yourself off and get back to it.

This isn't a competition. It isn't about how fast you are able to make the change. It doesn't matter what your neighbor is doing or even what they think about what you are doing. This is a personal journey that has a rippling effect on your environment and in turn everyone else's environment too. It doesn't matter if someone else is a hundred steps ahead of you in this journey to change or ten steps behind. We all start from where we are and move forward from there.

Today you brought your bags to the store, yesterday you bought the bags at the store. Tomorrow, you take your own glass, metal, paper, bamboo straw with you to the restaurant where you can simply say, "a glass of water, no straw".

Close to zero (low) waste isn't about perfectionism, it's about embracing the imperfection in practicing something that, when done well, will make the world a better space for everyone. You aren't perfect...I know I know, your mom said you were perfect, but you know moms. Being perfect is perfectly fine. But difficult to sustain. The higher the pedestal the harder the fall. We are all about what is sustainable. So being perfectly imperfect is perfectly fine too! We just have to be able to do it for the long haul. Things that won't make us feel like our lives aren't worth living. We are only trying to do the best we can in living our best lives, while ensuring the planet we live on continues to be able to supply us with the necessities needed for life. The planet provides everything we need, but not everything we want.

We just want to make every little bit count. Do our part without feeling that we are failures. You aren't a failure because you failed, failure occurs when you stop picking yourself back up.

"If you live in harmony with nature you will never be poor; if you live according to what others think, you will never be rich." Seneca, Letters from a Stoic

"One child, one teacher, one pen, and one book can change the world" -Malala Yousafzai

Chapter Nine

Make a difference

"One person can make a difference, and everyone should try."- John F. Kennedy

When we go to the store and that person snipes that parking space right out from under us, we get a little mad. That was one person changed your emotions if only for a moment. Just one person made some sort of impact on you for the briefest of moments. Because of that you might ignore the door greeter who cheerfully blurted out "Hello" to you as you walked in and right past them without even looking. That person that stole that parking spot right out from under you affected you, and you in turn affected that greeter. While this is an example of how one person can make a negative impact on us, what we want to do is make a positive impact on the world...one person at a time.

I have double deficit dyslexia, so school was hard for me. More accurately, English class was really hard for me. I read slowly, couldn't sound out words (hooked on Phonics didn't work for me) so I had to look up words in the dictionary and thesaurus to find a replacement word I could use in the sentence. Stress or lack of sleep causes stuttering and, what I call, word salad. My brain knows all the words I want to use but for some reason the space between my brain and my mouth the words were tossed like a salad and come out in some random nonsense order.

One person made a difference for me in school. I had an 8th grade speed reading teacher that knew my plight and still allowed me to join her class. She understood that I would fail based on the syllabus but we both knew that wasn't my bar for success. I wanted to be able to read faster than I currently did...I wanted to "read like a normal person". That's what I said. Normal, like I wasn't normal. That was my mindset.

That teacher could have graded me based on the syllabus and failed me, which would have held me back a year. But she took into consideration my disability, my goals, where I was starting from and at the end of that term gave me a D to pass. Where I ended up at the end of the marking term showed steady progress. I had increased my reading speed exponentially...I just still didn't speed read, but I read "like a normal person". That teacher passing me elevated my self-confidence instead of tearing it down. She didn't have to do that. She didn't have to let me in the class. She didn't have to pass me. But because she did, I went on to high school with a level of self-confidence that allowed me to remove my educational accommodations and still graduate. It gave me the confidence to do what I wanted to do. I eventually went on to get both a bachelor's and master's degree.

We are only limited by our imagination and tenacity. I basically failed that class, but I wasn't a failure because I did succeed in learning what I'm made of. I stood up, brushed myself off and kept on going.

Speaking of tenacity, Greta Thunberg! Now there is a kid who knows what she wants and lets it be known. She is one teenager that made a huge difference and got people talking. She realized the dangers of not doing anything about the climate would kill us all.

Greta started as a single person strike from school in front of her Swedish parliament building protesting the need for climate policy change. She sparked a revolution in our youth across the globe. She opened the communication lines between those that make the policies and those who have to live with them. She was invited to speak in front of the world's leaders at the United Nations

Climate Action Summit in 2019. Greta's passion for the environment and her steadfastness at the need for change helped name her "Time's Person of the Year 2019", but more importantly, she changed who was at the table in making climate policy changes. She is just one person that sparked an entire movement in the next generation.

One person can, and does, make a difference! While you might look at your recycling bin and see that you are only sending about a ton of recyclables to the recycling center a year and they process 300 tons in a year, that one ton is the difference between finishing a bale for sale and not having enough material. Let's look at it in smaller terms. You've been saving those random pennies on the ground you find in the center console of your car, and you go to buy a lemonade from the neighbor kid, but you're short 11 cents...but wait, your car pennies are 11 cents!! It made a difference, and it was only a penny every few weeks.

Never downplay your role in making a difference in someone's life or in the life of the planet.

"Recycling and packaging businesses are changing all of those things because that's what consumers want." – Jerry Greenfield, Co-founder of Ben & Jerry's Ice Cream

Making Change with your voice (vote and dollar)

The easiest way to make a change is with how you spend your hard-earned cash. I'm not talking about special interest lobbying, or contributing to some political campaign, I'm talking about what you buy or don't buy and who you buy from. Plus, which companies you invest in for your 401K or IRA. Also, who you vote for as your elected officials at the local, state and federal levels.

We will start with who you invest in.

The fossil fuel industry accounts for 10% of the carbon emissions and the big four claim that they are working towards net-zero carbon but their investments and actions say otherwise.... BP, Chevron, ExxonMobil and Shell[7]. While the world is in freefall with recessions and inflation, they continue to rob us of our money and bring in quarter after quarter of profits.

---

[7] Accusations of 'greenwashing' by big oil companies are well-founded, a new study finds. Joe Herandez. Feb. 2022. https://www.npr.org/2022/02/16/1081119920/greenwashing-oil-companies

Walmart, Home Depot, Amazon, and Nike are the worst overseas shipping polluters out there for 2020[8]. Just one example, Walmart generates more greenhouse gasses than a coal plant does in a year! They all have sustainability claims and goals of reducing their carbon footprint over the next 25-30 years...so we will have to keep an eye on them to see if they can get off the list.

Those companies that are living up to their claims of being environmentally friendly are: Patagonia, Seventh Generation, A Good Company, Pela, Dr. Bonner's, Allbirds, Tentree, Aspiration, Mud Jeans, and Grove Collaboration. [9] They might not necessarily be huge

------

[8] Walmart, Target, and Amazon are among the biggest corporate polluters thanks to overseas shipping. HannahTowey. July 2021. https://www.businessinsider.com/walmart-target-amazon-among-biggest-maritime-polluters-overseas-shipping-impact-report-2021-7

[9] https://growensemble.com/environmentally-friendly-companies/

brand names now, but they are on the rise.

"It's not what you have but who you are that counts."

— Frank Sonnenberg

Next, let's look at the companies that have given to federal politicians and then to the politicians that have taken the money. We have to decide if they are thinking and working for us or for someone else; who's values and priorities match our own.

<u>Top companies that have given</u>

Koch Industries—$5.96m

Conoco Phillips-$5.87m

Occidental Petroleum-$3.98m

Chevron Corp- $3.94m

Exxon Mobil- $3.72m

Top ten politicians that have taken money from the oil and gas

Manchin, Joe (D-WV)- $694k

McCarthy, Kevin (R-CA)- $433k

Lankford, James (R-OK)- $371k

Pfluger, August (R-TX)- $336k

Murkowski, Lisa (R-AK)- $316k[10]

If these politicians don't line up with your values and priorities, then it's time to not elect them to yet another term.

You shouldn't just vote party line; you should look at where your values lay and research the candidates (federal and local) to see who lines up closest to your values.

Where we buy. It's a good idea to look for bulk, refill locations. Now if you are in New Jersey, you have a fantastic option at the Dry Goods

---

[10] Open secrets

Refillery or in Florida you have Bulk Nation. Most Whole Foods, Sprouts, and Wincos all have some bulk food areas in the stores. It's not as much as a store that is specifically for that but it's a good start.

If you aren't near any of those options, then when you buy make sure to choose items with no or little packaging. When you go to the grocery store, try to buy your produce without plastic wrapping and don't use the plastic bags to keep them all together. You can go to a "u-pick" farm or farmer's market.

I spend a little extra and check with the butcher for our meat because it doesn't come in foam and plastic packaging. But I have to confess I don't use the deli for my lunch meat because the plastic that they put the meat and cheese in isn't as easily recyclable; plus, I like to use the plastic containers the lunch meat comes in as my Tupperware, so I reuse that container for a few years before it needs to be recycled.

When I have items I don't need, I look to friends and family first to see if they need it. I like to buy second hand when possible and live with the "one in one out" rule. My dollars are given to charities that align with my values (4Oceans, the Nature Conservancy, National Wildlife Federation).

*"Knowledge is power.
Sharing knowledge is the key
to unlocking that power." —
Martin Uzochukwu Ugwu*

Much like that question, "what one person can do?", if we don't share what we know nothing can change. We need to take time to talk about what changes we have or are going to make. But it's equally important to talk about why we made them.

"The earth is what we all have in common"- Wendell Berry

A good example of how not to talk about what you are doing or what you have learned is vegans screaming "meat is murder". Of course, it is the animal was alive and now it's not. A better way to get people to hear what you have to say is to calmly explain why meat is murder. The amount of energy, resources, and time that is put into raising an animal for only 18 months and then the inhumane way that they are killed, chickens heads cut off while they are still alive, a pig with a bolt in its head, baby cows that can't run or move so their meat stays tender, that might get someone thinking about if they could at least start with a meatless Monday to help reduce the amount of animal flesh they consume.

When someone shares with you what they know, YOU now know something new. What you do with that new information is entirely up to you. Do you share that information with the next person or keep it to yourself? Sharing is Caring!!

"There is no wealth like knowledge, and no poverty like ignorance." Buddha

Use that new information and make something great! Make those changes that will help you and your environment. But I have to say don't make changes because someone else told you to, it won't last. You have to want to make the changes, and I hope that you do want to make some of the changes we have talked about. Make sure that any changes you make are aligned with who you are, it will make them easier to do. Challenge your beliefs and values. Ask yourself why you have those values and beliefs? Are they still working for you? Are you still the same person? Did your values and beliefs grow with you over the years?

You can join meet ups of like-minded people to get to know others in your area that have the same values and come together to advocate for changes in your local area. Or start a nonprofit that helps with some issue in your area that you would like to change. Maybe you want to have a straw ban or single use plastic bag ban in your city/town. Maybe you want to help the homeless find meaningful work and housing. Maybe you want to stop the grocery stores from locking the dumpster behind their stores or donate all food that they would have thrown away.

Explain to people why you have made the change. The change is great but the knowledge of why and how is just as important. If the meteorologist didn't forecast rain, would we actually have an umbrella with us all the time? Probably not. If the doctor didn't tell us that our cholesterol levels were dangerously high, would we cut out the pound of butter? Probably not. We can't change what we don't have any idea about. And when we are told, we usually want to know why and how something is the way it is. But I am a "why" kid, I just want to know, I need to know the why of something. I'm not saying you need to go door to door like a vacuum salesman or a missionary, I'm just saying, find ways to bring it up in conversations.

"I believe our biggest issue is the same biggest issue that the whole world is facing, and that's habitat destruction."

-Steve Irwin

Chapter ten

Putting it all together

"Be the change you want to see in the world" -Mahatma Gandhi (paraphrased)

Little things you do that will make a bigger difference than you ever thought they could, did so, not because you did them perfectly, but that you did them consistently.

Waking up at 5 am three days of the week isn't going to change you into a morning person, but doing it every day for three months will make it a whole lot harder to sleep in.

Consistency is what's going to make the change stick. But let's look at some of the things we might want to change.

- Make a list of your beliefs and values.
    - Do they still resonate with you?
- Keep a journal of your daily habits.
    - Are there any you'd like to change?

- Sit with yourself and be mindful of your feelings and thoughts.
- Make a checklist of what you want to change.
- Go for the low hanging fruit first.
  - Reduce using single use bags to carry things that you are just going to throw away empty when you get home.
  - Reduce the use of single use straws, say "no" to the straw or bring your own.
  - Buy only what you need, when you need it.
  - Follow the Rs on what to do with something when

it's time to leave you has arrived.

- ○ Reduce your water usage:
    - ■ Fix the leaks.
    - ■ Keep your irrigation water usage to a minimum.
    - ■ Reduce the length of your shower.
- Talk about the environment, climate change, and your part in it all, with your family and friends.
- Make new friends that have the same values and interests as you.
- Talk with people that don't think like you.

- Join environmental organizations.

Remember, a baby doesn't go from laying there without rolling over to winning a marathon...there are a lot of steps in between there!

Lifestyle Change

Going green, zero waste, environmentally conscious are all lifestyle changes, not just words used to make us feel better or sound like we care. Throughout this book we have talked about <u>why it's important</u> to make the changes and <u>how to</u> take those first steps.

Change is hard but if it's something you want to do, you'll push through.

Just remember to Focus on The Big Picture. Why are you doing the changes?

Set realistic and achievable goals. Use SMART to make the changes.

Specific, Measurable, Achievable, Relevant, and Time-Bound

Example: reduce plastic bags (Specific)

There are less bags in your bags of bags (Measurable)

Not that hard to not grab them (Achievable)

Reducing the bags is good for the landfill and the ocean (Relevant)

By the end of next month, I will only use my reusable bags (Time-bound)

Create daily routines. Every morning fill a water bottle with something to drink on the way to work so you aren't tempted to stop at Starbucks for a drink.

Make habits you can keep. Remember sustainability is the key. Doing it once is nice, doing it all the time is hard, doing it most of the time is sustainable.

Use the technique of habit stacking. Start with one item and build from there. Go for the "low hanging fruit" first and then slowly add another habit and another till you reach the level you can sustain.

Share the journey. Everything's better with a buddy. If you can share what you have learned with others, they can make the change with you and the two of you can hold one another accountable. It works for the gym, why not for the planet.

Track your progress. Remember that "ta done" list.

Make a list of all the changes you want to make. Tick them off as you try them. Journal about which ones stick, and why. AND which one's don't stick, and why. Failure is as important as success to help us learn.

Balance in all things. Sustainability!!!

This book was never intended to be the end all of what to do, but a launching pad to help you start to do small things that will add up over time and with the increase of more people doing it change is possible.

Remember, **"We don't need a handful of people doing zero waste perfectly. We need millions of people doing it imperfectly."** Thank you Anne Marie Bonneau.

Our children and our children's children need us to step up and do what we can to ensure they have a world to live in, to breathe, to frolic in, and to pass on to the next generations so our species doesn't go extinct.

"Life is too short to bullshit."
— Fakeer Ishavardas

I tried not to bullshit you! Everything I suggested are things that I have done, am doing, try to remember to do on the daily. I'm not perfect, which is perfect! I am perfectly imperfect at doing my part. I still forget my reusable bags in the car and sometimes at the house, but thanks to my purse bags I have at least three small reusable bags to use to reduce the number of single use plastic ones I have to use. I still get popcorn and a soda at the movies. I still ride alone in my car to and from work five days a week.

But I do try to do all my errands on the way home from work, so I don't have to go out again on the weekends or after I've gotten home. I wear my jeans at least twice before washing them, my towel remains on the towel bar for three full shower days, my toothbrush is bamboo and I take a 5-minute shower (except for hair washing days...then it's eight minutes). I make sure that when I buy something it's preferably in metal packaging or fiber so it can be recyclable in my curbside bin. I have learned which items that I can do, and which ones are outside of my conscious ability to remember. The average American creates almost 5 lbs. of trash a day. I'm not at zero but I am at around one pound or less a day. So even the small things I am doing are making a difference. I can see it, it's measurable, and it's attainable on a sustainable level for me.

"Everything is within your power,
and your power is within you."
— Janice Trachtman

If the pandemic of 2019 taught us anything it's that Mother Nature can recover quickly if given the opportunity. The world shut down for one year and the people of India could see the Himalayas for the first time in a generation. The people in China were wearing masks for the pandemic but not because of air quality. The sea turtles were able to get to and lay their eggs on the beaches without wading through a shore filled with trash. The pandemic moved the overshoot day back 21 days. Now I'm not saying that the pandemic was a brilliant way to help the planet (it's not sustainable for us) but it shows that changes can be made to make a difference.

Here is a list of things you might have known are compostable from around the house. Be sure to use the right items in the correct types of bins. Some items won't work for worms. The list is broken down by both Greens (Nitrogen) or Browns (Carbon) and by area of the house.

From the Kitchen

Greens:
1. Food Scraps
2. Stale beer, wine, pumpkin, sunflower or sesame seeds
3. Avocado pits
4. Moldy cheese (in moderation)
5. Melted ice cream (in moderation)
6. Old jelly, jam, or preserves

Browns:
7. Paper napkins, towels, paper and cardboard
8. The crumbs you sweep off of the counters and floors
9. Stale breads, chips, crackers, cereal
10. Crumbs from the bottom of snack food packaging

11. Wine corks (chop up so they decompose faster)
12. Toothpicks and bamboo skewers
13. Egg shells (crushed)
14. Coffee filters
15. Tea bags if natural materials

From the Bathroom

Greens:
1. Menstrual blood
2. Urine

Browns:
3. Used facial tissues
4. Hair from your hairbrush
5. Trimmings from an electric razor and nail clipper
6. Toilet paper rolls (shredded)
7. Old loofahs (cut up, natural only)
8. 100% cotton cotton balls and swabs
9. 100% cotton tampons and sanitary pads (including used)
10. Cardboard tampon applicators

From the Laundry Room

All Browns:
1. Dryer lint (from 100% natural fabrics only!)

2. Old cotton and wool clothing, jeans (ripped or cut into small pieces) and scraps

From the Office

All Browns:

1. Bills and other plain paper documents (shredded)
2. Envelopes (shredded, minus the plastic window)
3. Pencil shavings
4. Sticky notes
5. Old business cards

Other Areas Around the House

Greens:

1. Leaves and flowers from houseplants and arrangements
2. Grass clippings

Browns:

3. "Dust bunnies" from wood and tile floors
4. Contents of your dustpan (pick out any inorganic stuff, like pennies and Legos)
5. Crumbs from under your couch cushions (again, pick out any inorganic stuff)
6. Paper
7. Burlap sacks, ropes, and twine (cut or torn into small pieces)
8. Used matches

9. Ashes from untreated wood burned in the fireplace, grill, or outdoor fire pits (in very small amounts)
10. Dead autumn leaves
11. Sawdust (from plain wood that has NOT been pressure-treated, stained or painted)

Party and Holiday Supplies

Greens:

1. Jack O'lanterns (smashed)

Browns:

2. Wrapping paper rolls (cut into smaller pieces)
3. Paper table cloths (shredded or torn into smaller pieces)
4. Crepe paper streamers (shredded)
5. Latex balloons (Make sure they are latex!)
6. Those hay bales you used as part of your outdoor fall decor (broken apart)
7. Natural holiday wreaths (chop up with pruners first)
8. Christmas trees (chop up with pruners first, or use a wood chipper, if you have one...)
9. Evergreen garlands (chop up with pruners first)

Pet-Related

Greens:

1. Droppings and bedding from your herbivorous pet rabbit, gerbil, hamster, etc. (Do NOT use dog or cat poop.)
2. Newspaper/droppings from the bottom of the bird or snake cage
3. Horse, cow or goat manure

Browns:

4. Feathers
5. Alfalfa hay or pellets (usually fed to rabbits, gerbils, etc.)
6. Dry dog or cat food, fish pellets
7. Fur from the dog or cat brush